MY ESSENTIAL OIL RECIPES

THIS BOOK BELONGS TO

_____

_____

_____

CONTACT DETAILS

_____

_____

_____

Dedication

This Essential Oils Blank Recipe Book is dedicated to all the people out there who love to make their own essential oil recipes and document their findings in the process.

You are my inspiration for producing books and I'm honored to be a part of keeping all of your Essential Oils notes and records organized.

This journal notebook will help you record your details about tracking your oils recipes.

Thoughtfully put together with these sections to record: Favorite Oils, Dilution Ratios, Safe For Children, Inventory, & Blank Recipe Pages.

How to Use this Book

The purpose of this book is to keep all of your Essential Oils Blank Recipe Book notes all in one place. It will help keep you organized.

This Essential Oils Blank Recipe Book will allow you to accurately document every detail about your recipes.

Here are examples of the prompts for you to fill in and write about your experience in this book:

1. Favorite Oil

2. Dilution Ratios

3. Safe Essential Oils For Children

4. Inventory

5. Recipe Pages

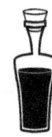 # MY FAVORITE OILS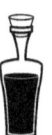

DILUTION RATIOS

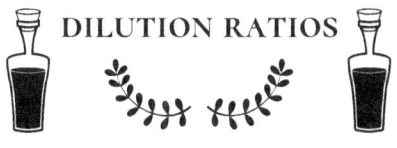

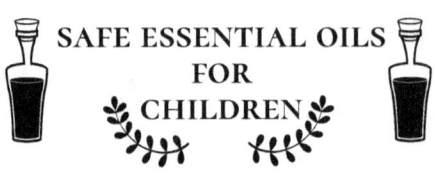

SAFE ESSENTIAL OILS FOR CHILDREN

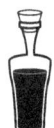   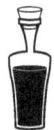

ESSENTIAL OILS INVENTORY

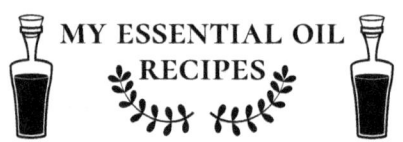
MY ESSENTIAL OIL RECIPES

OIL NAME

◯◯◯◯◯◯

BENEFITS
_____
_____
_____
_____

NOTES
_____
_____
_____
_____

OIL NAME

◯◯◯◯◯◯

BENEFITS
_____
_____
_____
_____

NOTES
_____
_____
_____
_____

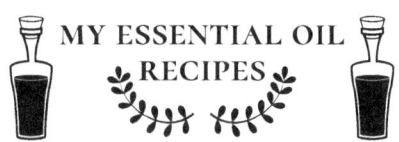
MY ESSENTIAL OIL RECIPES

OIL NAME

BENEFITS
_____
_____
_____
_____

NOTES
_____
_____
_____
_____

OIL NAME

BENEFITS
_____
_____
_____
_____

NOTES
_____
_____
_____
_____

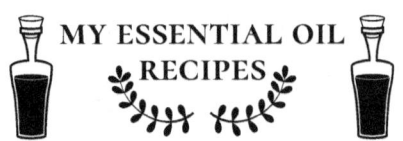

MY ESSENTIAL OIL RECIPES

OIL NAME

○○○○○○

BENEFITS
_____
_____
_____
_____

NOTES
_____
_____
_____
_____

OIL NAME

○○○○○○

BENEFITS
_____
_____
_____
_____

NOTES
_____
_____
_____
_____

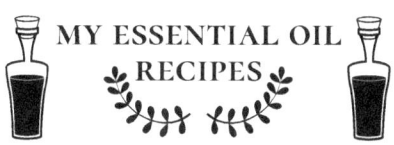
MY ESSENTIAL OIL RECIPES

OIL NAME

BENEFITS
_____
_____
_____
_____

NOTES
_____
_____
_____
_____

OIL NAME

BENEFITS
_____
_____
_____
_____

NOTES
_____
_____
_____
_____

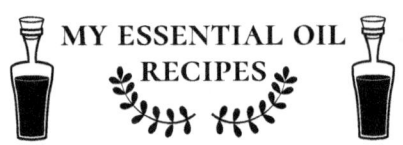

MY ESSENTIAL OIL RECIPES

OIL NAME

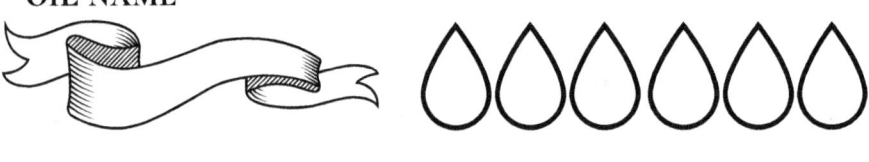

BENEFITS

_____
_____
_____
_____

NOTES

_____
_____
_____
_____

OIL NAME

BENEFITS

_____
_____
_____
_____

NOTES

_____
_____
_____
_____

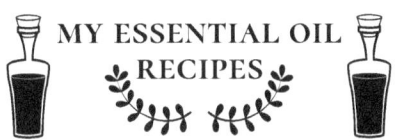

MY ESSENTIAL OIL RECIPES

OIL NAME

BENEFITS

NOTES

OIL NAME

BENEFITS

NOTES

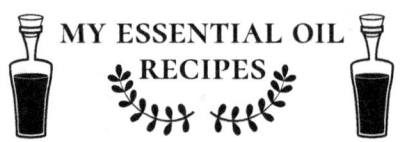

MY ESSENTIAL OIL RECIPES

OIL NAME

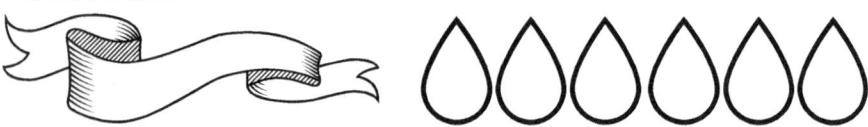

BENEFITS

_____
_____
_____
_____

NOTES

_____
_____
_____
_____

OIL NAME

BENEFITS

_____
_____
_____
_____

NOTES

_____
_____
_____
_____

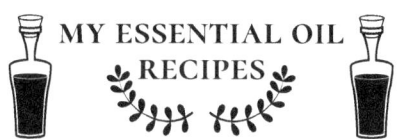

MY ESSENTIAL OIL RECIPES

OIL NAME

BENEFITS
_____
_____
_____

NOTES
_____
_____
_____

OIL NAME

BENEFITS
_____
_____
_____

NOTES
_____
_____
_____

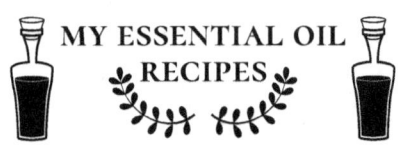

MY ESSENTIAL OIL RECIPES

OIL NAME

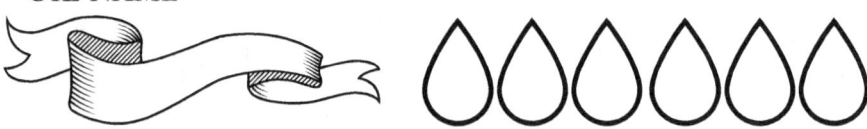

BENEFITS
_____
_____
_____
_____

NOTES
_____
_____
_____
_____

OIL NAME

BENEFITS
_____
_____
_____
_____

NOTES
_____
_____
_____
_____

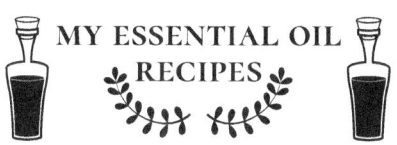

MY ESSENTIAL OIL RECIPES

OIL NAME

BENEFITS
_____
_____
_____
_____

NOTES
_____
_____
_____
_____

OIL NAME

BENEFITS
_____
_____
_____
_____

NOTES
_____
_____
_____
_____

MY ESSENTIAL OIL RECIPES

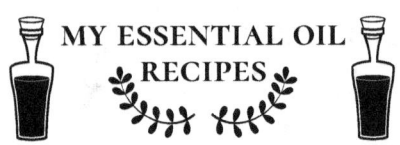

OIL NAME

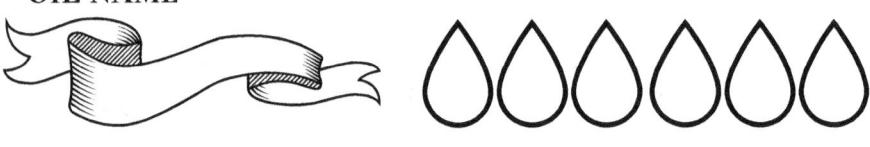

BENEFITS

_____
_____
_____

NOTES

_____
_____
_____

OIL NAME

BENEFITS

_____
_____
_____

NOTES

_____
_____
_____

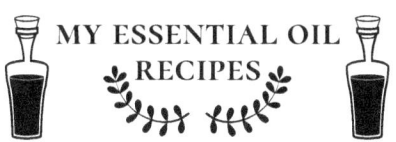

MY ESSENTIAL OIL RECIPES

OIL NAME

BENEFITS

NOTES

OIL NAME

BENEFITS

NOTES

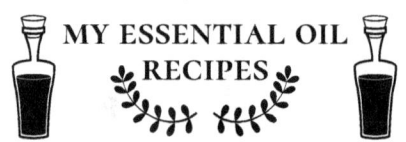
MY ESSENTIAL OIL RECIPES

OIL NAME

◊◊◊◊◊◊

BENEFITS

_____
_____
_____

NOTES

_____
_____
_____

OIL NAME

◊◊◊◊◊◊

BENEFITS

_____
_____
_____

NOTES

_____
_____
_____

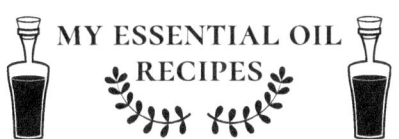

MY ESSENTIAL OIL RECIPES

OIL NAME

BENEFITS

NOTES

OIL NAME

BENEFITS

NOTES

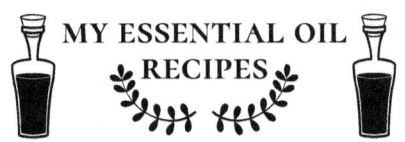

MY ESSENTIAL OIL RECIPES

OIL NAME

BENEFITS

NOTES

OIL NAME

BENEFITS

NOTES

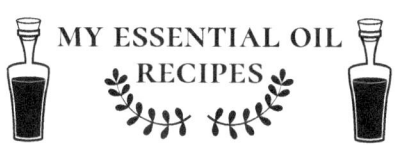

MY ESSENTIAL OIL RECIPES

OIL NAME

◊◊◊◊◊◊

BENEFITS

NOTES

OIL NAME

◊◊◊◊◊◊

BENEFITS

NOTES

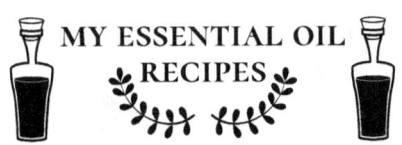

MY ESSENTIAL OIL RECIPES

OIL NAME

◯ ◯ ◯ ◯ ◯ ◯

BENEFITS

_____
_____
_____

NOTES

_____
_____
_____

OIL NAME

◯ ◯ ◯ ◯ ◯ ◯

BENEFITS

_____
_____
_____

NOTES

_____
_____
_____

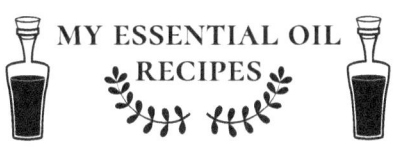

MY ESSENTIAL OIL RECIPES

OIL NAME

◇◇◇◇◇◇

BENEFITS

_____
_____
_____

NOTES

_____
_____
_____

OIL NAME

◇◇◇◇◇◇

BENEFITS

_____
_____
_____

NOTES

_____
_____
_____

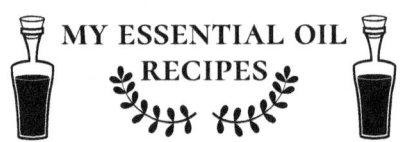

MY ESSENTIAL OIL RECIPES

OIL NAME

BENEFITS
_____
_____
_____

NOTES
_____
_____
_____
_____

OIL NAME

BENEFITS
_____
_____
_____

NOTES
_____
_____
_____
_____

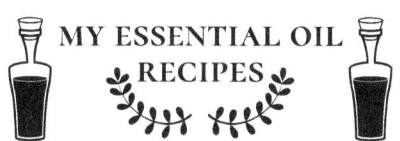

MY ESSENTIAL OIL RECIPES

OIL NAME

BENEFITS

NOTES

OIL NAME

BENEFITS

NOTES

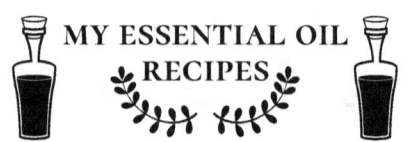

MY ESSENTIAL OIL RECIPES

OIL NAME

BENEFITS

NOTES

OIL NAME

BENEFITS

NOTES

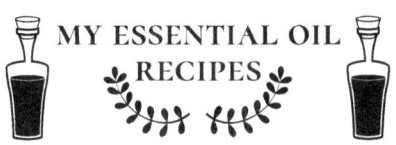

MY ESSENTIAL OIL RECIPES

OIL NAME

BENEFITS

_____
_____
_____

NOTES

_____
_____
_____

OIL NAME

BENEFITS

_____
_____
_____

NOTES

_____
_____
_____

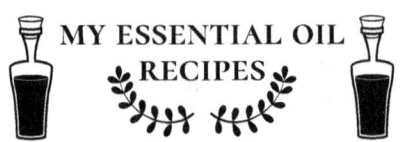

MY ESSENTIAL OIL RECIPES

OIL NAME

BENEFITS

NOTES

OIL NAME

BENEFITS

NOTES

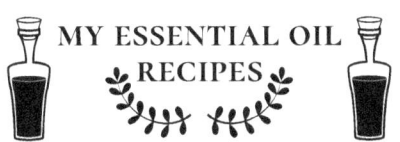

MY ESSENTIAL OIL RECIPES

OIL NAME

BENEFITS

NOTES

OIL NAME

BENEFITS

NOTES

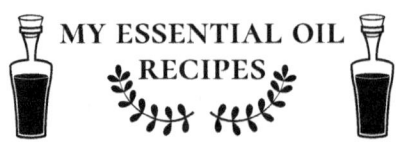

MY ESSENTIAL OIL RECIPES

OIL NAME

〇〇〇〇〇〇

BENEFITS

_____
_____
_____
_____

NOTES

_____
_____
_____
_____

OIL NAME

〇〇〇〇〇〇

BENEFITS

_____
_____
_____
_____

NOTES

_____
_____
_____
_____

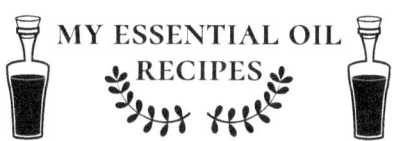

MY ESSENTIAL OIL RECIPES

OIL NAME

BENEFITS

NOTES

OIL NAME

BENEFITS

NOTES

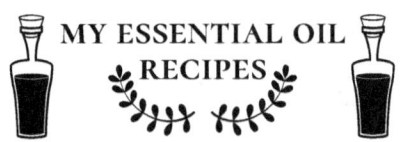

MY ESSENTIAL OIL RECIPES

OIL NAME

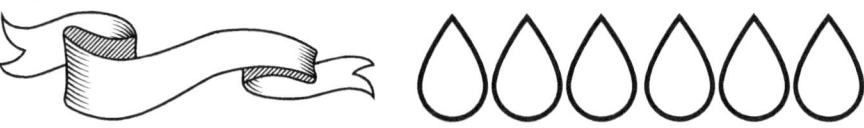

BENEFITS

_____
_____
_____
_____

NOTES

_____
_____
_____
_____

OIL NAME

BENEFITS

_____
_____
_____
_____

NOTES

_____
_____
_____
_____

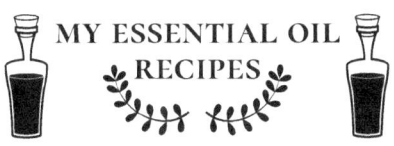
MY ESSENTIAL OIL RECIPES

OIL NAME

BENEFITS

_____
_____
_____

NOTES

_____
_____
_____

OIL NAME

BENEFITS

_____
_____
_____

NOTES

_____
_____
_____

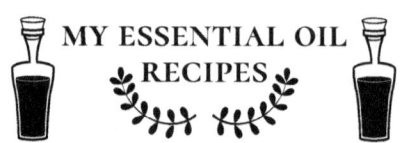

MY ESSENTIAL OIL RECIPES

OIL NAME

BENEFITS
_____
_____
_____
_____

NOTES
_____
_____
_____
_____

OIL NAME

BENEFITS
_____
_____
_____
_____

NOTES
_____
_____
_____
_____

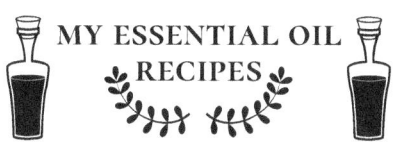
MY ESSENTIAL OIL RECIPES

OIL NAME

BENEFITS

NOTES

OIL NAME

BENEFITS

NOTES

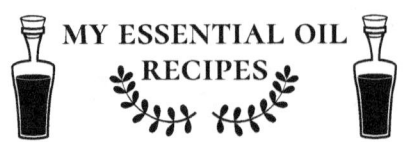

MY ESSENTIAL OIL RECIPES

OIL NAME

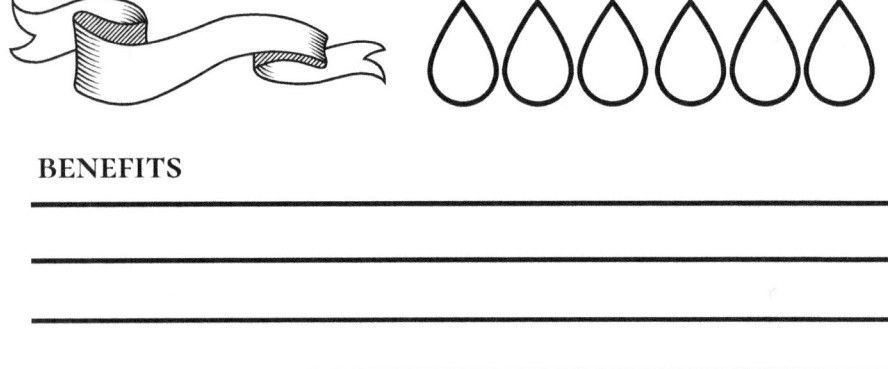

BENEFITS

_____
_____
_____

NOTES

_____
_____
_____
_____

OIL NAME

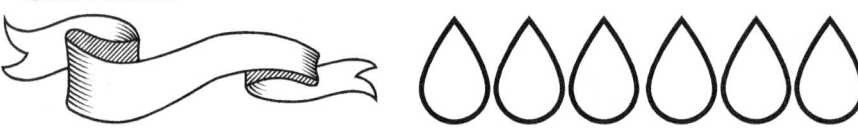

BENEFITS

_____
_____
_____

NOTES

_____
_____
_____
_____

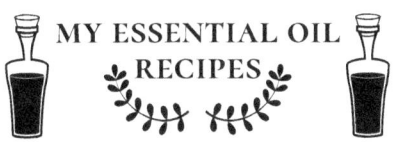

MY ESSENTIAL OIL RECIPES

OIL NAME

BENEFITS
_____
_____
_____

NOTES
_____
_____
_____

OIL NAME

BENEFITS
_____
_____
_____

NOTES
_____
_____
_____

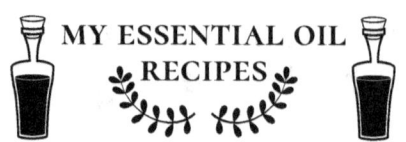

MY ESSENTIAL OIL RECIPES

OIL NAME

◯ ◯ ◯ ◯ ◯ ◯

BENEFITS

_____
_____
_____
_____

NOTES

_____
_____
_____
_____

OIL NAME

◯ ◯ ◯ ◯ ◯ ◯

BENEFITS

_____
_____
_____
_____

NOTES

_____
_____
_____
_____

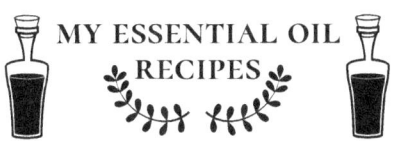
MY ESSENTIAL OIL RECIPES

OIL NAME

BENEFITS
_____
_____
_____

NOTES
_____
_____
_____

OIL NAME

BENEFITS
_____
_____
_____

NOTES
_____
_____
_____

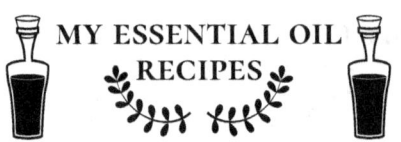
MY ESSENTIAL OIL RECIPES

OIL NAME

○○○○○○

BENEFITS
_____
_____
_____
_____

NOTES
_____
_____
_____
_____

OIL NAME

○○○○○○

BENEFITS
_____
_____
_____
_____

NOTES
_____
_____
_____
_____

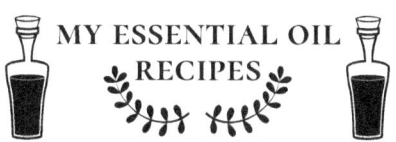

MY ESSENTIAL OIL RECIPES

OIL NAME

BENEFITS

NOTES

OIL NAME

BENEFITS

NOTES

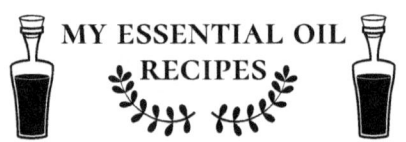

MY ESSENTIAL OIL RECIPES

OIL NAME

◊ ◊ ◊ ◊ ◊ ◊

BENEFITS
_____
_____
_____
_____

NOTES
_____
_____
_____
_____

OIL NAME

◊ ◊ ◊ ◊ ◊ ◊

BENEFITS
_____
_____
_____
_____

NOTES
_____
_____
_____
_____

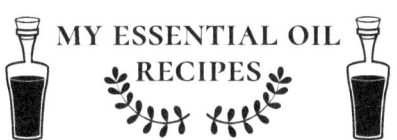
MY ESSENTIAL OIL RECIPES

OIL NAME

BENEFITS

NOTES

OIL NAME

BENEFITS

NOTES

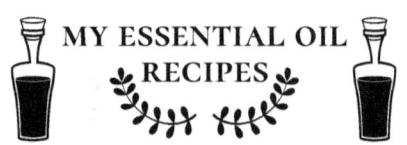
MY ESSENTIAL OIL RECIPES

OIL NAME

BENEFITS

NOTES

OIL NAME

BENEFITS

NOTES

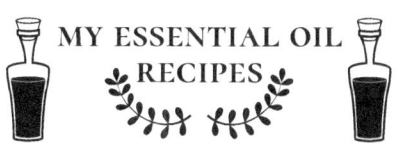

MY ESSENTIAL OIL RECIPES

OIL NAME

BENEFITS

_____
_____
_____
_____

NOTES

_____
_____
_____
_____

OIL NAME

BENEFITS

_____
_____
_____
_____

NOTES

_____
_____
_____
_____

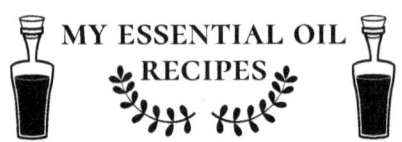

MY ESSENTIAL OIL RECIPES

OIL NAME

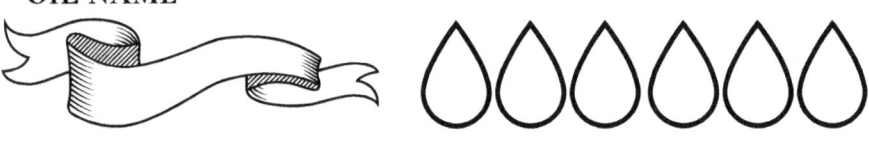

BENEFITS

_____
_____
_____
_____

NOTES

_____
_____
_____
_____

OIL NAME

BENEFITS

_____
_____
_____
_____

NOTES

_____
_____
_____
_____

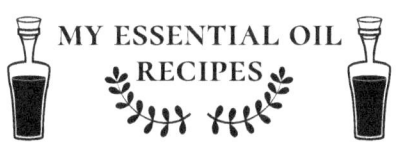

MY ESSENTIAL OIL RECIPES

OIL NAME

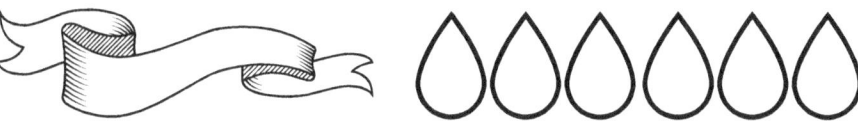

BENEFITS

_____
_____
_____
_____

NOTES

_____
_____
_____
_____

OIL NAME

BENEFITS

_____
_____
_____
_____

NOTES

_____
_____
_____
_____

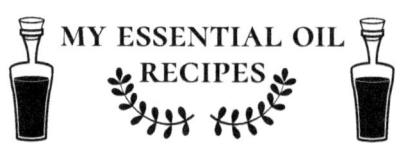
MY ESSENTIAL OIL RECIPES

OIL NAME

BENEFITS
_____
_____
_____
_____

NOTES
_____
_____
_____
_____

OIL NAME

BENEFITS
_____
_____
_____
_____

NOTES
_____
_____
_____
_____

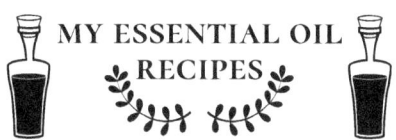
MY ESSENTIAL OIL RECIPES

OIL NAME

BENEFITS

NOTES

OIL NAME

BENEFITS

NOTES

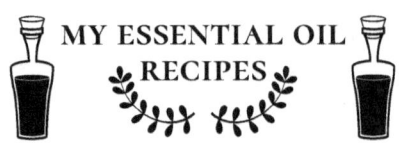
MY ESSENTIAL OIL RECIPES

OIL NAME

○○○○○○

BENEFITS
_____
_____
_____
_____

NOTES
_____
_____
_____
_____

OIL NAME

○○○○○○

BENEFITS
_____
_____
_____
_____

NOTES
_____
_____
_____
_____

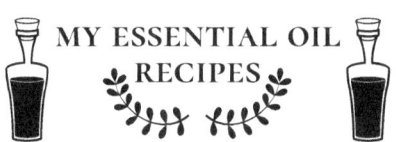
MY ESSENTIAL OIL RECIPES

OIL NAME

BENEFITS
_____
_____
_____
_____

NOTES
_____
_____
_____
_____

OIL NAME

BENEFITS
_____
_____
_____
_____

NOTES
_____
_____
_____
_____

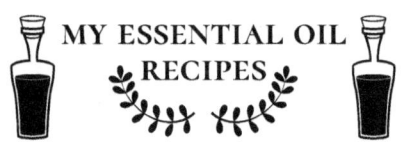

MY ESSENTIAL OIL RECIPES

OIL NAME

BENEFITS

NOTES

OIL NAME

BENEFITS

NOTES

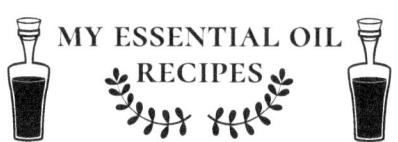

MY ESSENTIAL OIL RECIPES

OIL NAME

BENEFITS

NOTES

OIL NAME

BENEFITS

NOTES

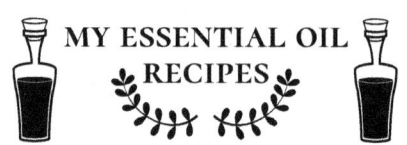

MY ESSENTIAL OIL RECIPES

OIL NAME

△△△△△△

BENEFITS

_____
_____
_____
_____

NOTES

_____
_____
_____
_____

OIL NAME

△△△△△△

BENEFITS

_____
_____
_____
_____

NOTES

_____
_____
_____
_____

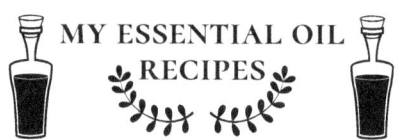

MY ESSENTIAL OIL RECIPES

OIL NAME

BENEFITS

NOTES

OIL NAME

BENEFITS

NOTES

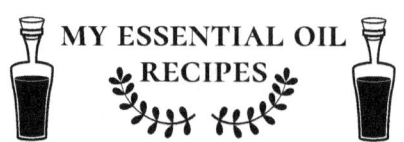

MY ESSENTIAL OIL RECIPES

OIL NAME

○○○○○○

BENEFITS

_____
_____
_____
_____

NOTES

_____
_____
_____
_____

OIL NAME

○○○○○○

BENEFITS

_____
_____
_____
_____

NOTES

_____
_____
_____
_____

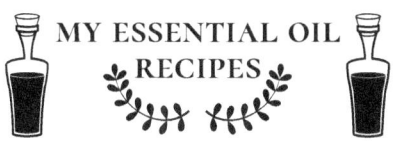
MY ESSENTIAL OIL RECIPES

OIL NAME

○○○○○○

BENEFITS
_____
_____
_____
_____

NOTES
_____
_____
_____
_____

OIL NAME

○○○○○○

BENEFITS
_____
_____
_____
_____

NOTES
_____
_____
_____
_____

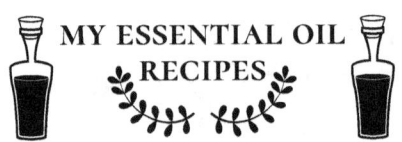

MY ESSENTIAL OIL RECIPES

OIL NAME

○○○○○○

BENEFITS

_____
_____
_____

NOTES

_____
_____
_____

OIL NAME

○○○○○○

BENEFITS

_____
_____
_____

NOTES

_____
_____
_____

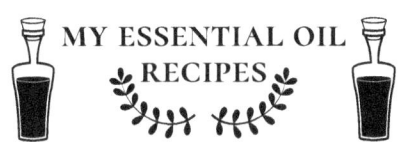

MY ESSENTIAL OIL RECIPES

OIL NAME

BENEFITS

NOTES

OIL NAME

BENEFITS

NOTES

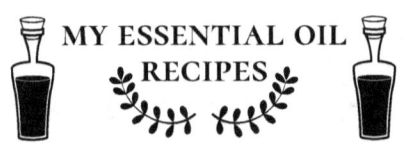

MY ESSENTIAL OIL RECIPES

OIL NAME

○○○○○○

BENEFITS

_____
_____
_____
_____

NOTES

_____
_____
_____
_____

OIL NAME

○○○○○○

BENEFITS

_____
_____
_____
_____

NOTES

_____
_____
_____
_____

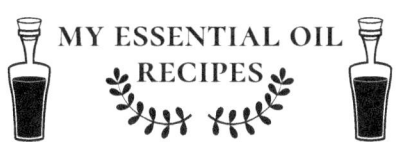

MY ESSENTIAL OIL RECIPES

OIL NAME

BENEFITS

NOTES

OIL NAME

BENEFITS

NOTES

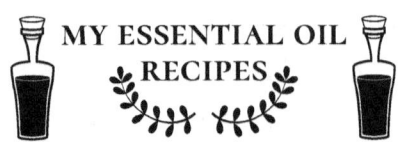
MY ESSENTIAL OIL RECIPES

OIL NAME

BENEFITS
_____
_____
_____
_____

NOTES
_____
_____
_____
_____

OIL NAME

BENEFITS
_____
_____
_____
_____

NOTES
_____
_____
_____
_____

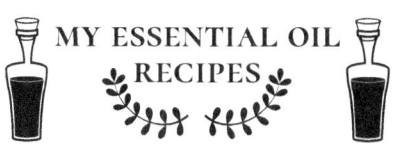

MY ESSENTIAL OIL RECIPES

OIL NAME

BENEFITS
_____
_____
_____

NOTES
_____
_____
_____

OIL NAME

BENEFITS
_____
_____
_____

NOTES
_____
_____
_____

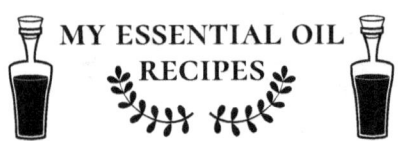
MY ESSENTIAL OIL RECIPES

OIL NAME

◯ ◯ ◯ ◯ ◯

BENEFITS
___
___
___
___

NOTES
___
___
___
___

OIL NAME

◯ ◯ ◯ ◯ ◯

BENEFITS
___
___
___
___

NOTES
___
___
___
___

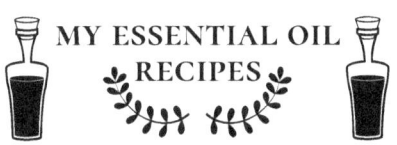

MY ESSENTIAL OIL RECIPES

OIL NAME

BENEFITS
_____
_____
_____
_____

NOTES
_____
_____
_____
_____

OIL NAME

BENEFITS
_____
_____
_____
_____

NOTES
_____
_____
_____
_____

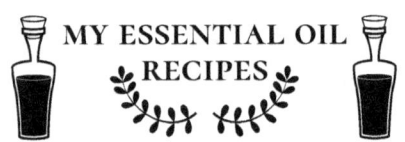

MY ESSENTIAL OIL RECIPES

OIL NAME

BENEFITS
_____
_____
_____

NOTES
_____
_____
_____

OIL NAME

BENEFITS
_____
_____
_____

NOTES
_____
_____
_____

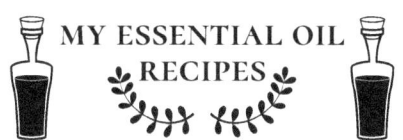

MY ESSENTIAL OIL RECIPES

OIL NAME

BENEFITS
_____
_____
_____
_____

NOTES
_____
_____
_____
_____
_____

OIL NAME

BENEFITS
_____
_____
_____
_____

NOTES
_____
_____
_____
_____
_____

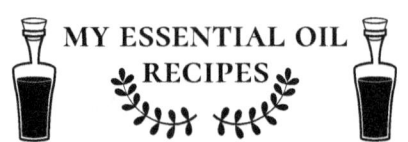
MY ESSENTIAL OIL RECIPES

OIL NAME

◊ ◊ ◊ ◊ ◊ ◊

BENEFITS
_____
_____
_____
_____

NOTES
_____
_____
_____
_____

OIL NAME

◊ ◊ ◊ ◊ ◊ ◊

BENEFITS
_____
_____
_____
_____

NOTES
_____
_____
_____
_____

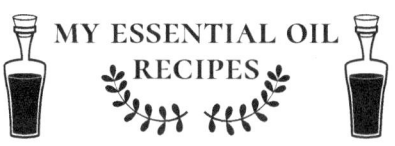

MY ESSENTIAL OIL RECIPES

OIL NAME

BENEFITS

NOTES

OIL NAME

BENEFITS

NOTES

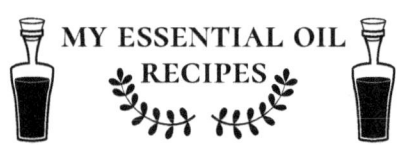

MY ESSENTIAL OIL RECIPES

OIL NAME

◊ ◊ ◊ ◊ ◊ ◊

BENEFITS
_____
_____
_____
_____

NOTES
_____
_____
_____
_____

OIL NAME

◊ ◊ ◊ ◊ ◊ ◊

BENEFITS
_____
_____
_____
_____

NOTES
_____
_____
_____
_____

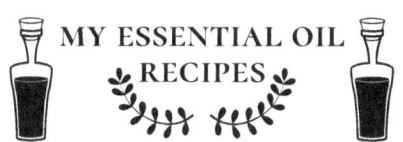

MY ESSENTIAL OIL RECIPES

OIL NAME

BENEFITS

_____
_____
_____
_____

NOTES

_____
_____
_____
_____

OIL NAME

BENEFITS

_____
_____
_____
_____

NOTES

_____
_____
_____
_____

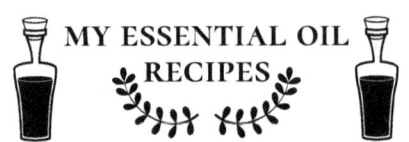

MY ESSENTIAL OIL RECIPES

OIL NAME

△△△△△△

BENEFITS
_____
_____
_____
_____

NOTES
_____
_____
_____
_____

OIL NAME

△△△△△△

BENEFITS
_____
_____
_____
_____

NOTES
_____
_____
_____
_____

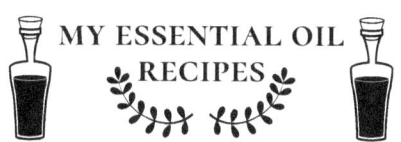

MY ESSENTIAL OIL RECIPES

OIL NAME

BENEFITS
_____
_____
_____
_____

NOTES
_____
_____
_____
_____

OIL NAME

BENEFITS
_____
_____
_____
_____

NOTES
_____
_____
_____
_____

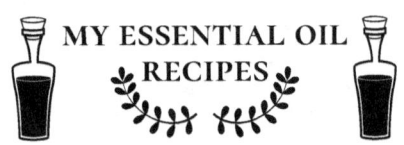

MY ESSENTIAL OIL RECIPES

OIL NAME

○○○○○○

BENEFITS

_____
_____
_____
_____

NOTES

_____
_____
_____
_____

OIL NAME

○○○○○○

BENEFITS

_____
_____
_____
_____

NOTES

_____
_____
_____
_____

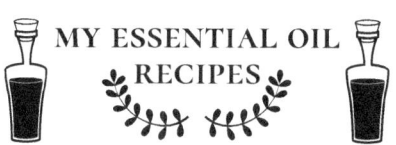

MY ESSENTIAL OIL RECIPES

OIL NAME

BENEFITS
_____
_____
_____
_____

NOTES
_____
_____
_____
_____

OIL NAME

BENEFITS
_____
_____
_____
_____

NOTES
_____
_____
_____
_____

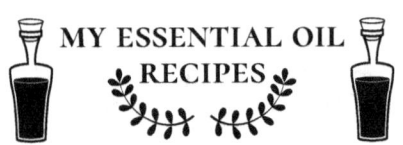
MY ESSENTIAL OIL RECIPES

OIL NAME

◯ ◯ ◯ ◯ ◯ ◯

BENEFITS
___
___
___

NOTES
___
___
___

OIL NAME

◯ ◯ ◯ ◯ ◯ ◯

BENEFITS
___
___
___

NOTES
___
___
___

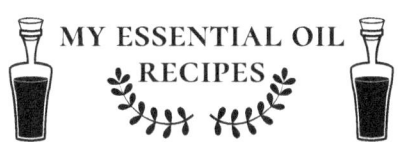

MY ESSENTIAL OIL RECIPES

OIL NAME

BENEFITS
_____
_____
_____
_____

NOTES
_____
_____
_____
_____

OIL NAME

BENEFITS
_____
_____
_____
_____

NOTES
_____
_____
_____
_____

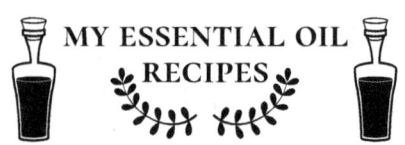

MY ESSENTIAL OIL RECIPES

OIL NAME

◯ ◯ ◯ ◯ ◯ ◯

BENEFITS
_____
_____
_____
_____

NOTES
_____
_____
_____
_____

OIL NAME

◯ ◯ ◯ ◯ ◯ ◯

BENEFITS
_____
_____
_____
_____

NOTES
_____
_____
_____
_____

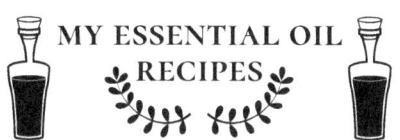
MY ESSENTIAL OIL RECIPES

OIL NAME

〇〇〇〇〇〇

BENEFITS
_____
_____
_____

NOTES
_____
_____
_____
_____

OIL NAME

〇〇〇〇〇〇

BENEFITS
_____
_____
_____

NOTES
_____
_____
_____
_____

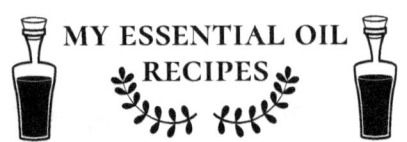
MY ESSENTIAL OIL RECIPES

OIL NAME

BENEFITS

NOTES

OIL NAME

BENEFITS

NOTES

MY ESSENTIAL OIL RECIPES

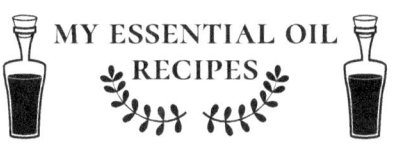

OIL NAME

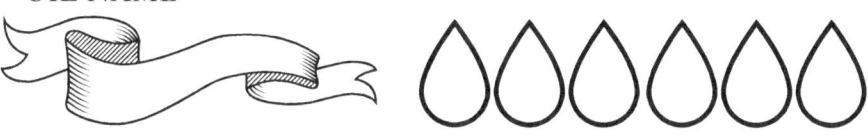

BENEFITS

_____
_____
_____

NOTES

_____
_____
_____

OIL NAME

BENEFITS

_____
_____
_____

NOTES

_____
_____
_____

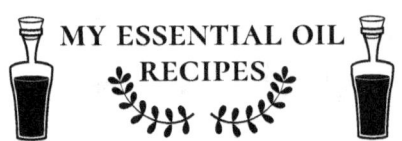

MY ESSENTIAL OIL RECIPES

OIL NAME

◯ ◯ ◯ ◯ ◯ ◯

BENEFITS
_____
_____
_____
_____

NOTES
_____
_____
_____
_____

OIL NAME

◯ ◯ ◯ ◯ ◯ ◯

BENEFITS
_____
_____
_____
_____

NOTES
_____
_____
_____
_____

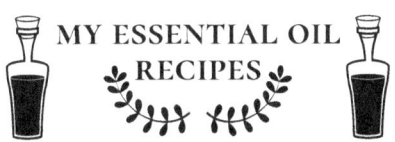

MY ESSENTIAL OIL RECIPES

OIL NAME

BENEFITS

NOTES

OIL NAME

BENEFITS

NOTES

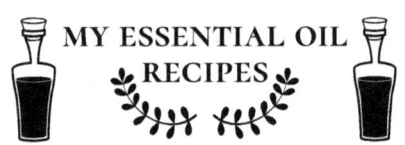

MY ESSENTIAL OIL RECIPES

OIL NAME

○○○○○○

BENEFITS

_____
_____
_____
_____

NOTES

_____
_____
_____
_____

OIL NAME

○○○○○○

BENEFITS

_____
_____
_____
_____

NOTES

_____
_____
_____
_____

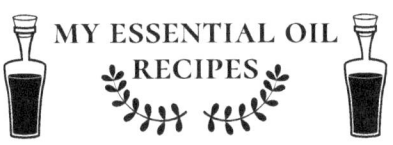

MY ESSENTIAL OIL RECIPES

OIL NAME

BENEFITS

NOTES

OIL NAME

BENEFITS

NOTES

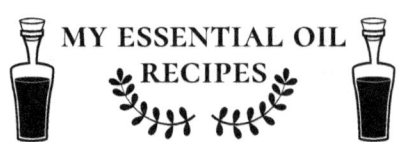
MY ESSENTIAL OIL RECIPES

OIL NAME

BENEFITS
_____
_____
_____
_____

NOTES
_____
_____
_____
_____

OIL NAME

BENEFITS
_____
_____
_____
_____

NOTES
_____
_____
_____
_____

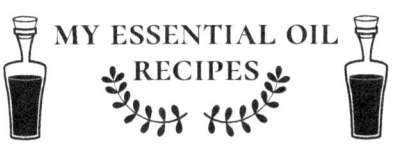

MY ESSENTIAL OIL RECIPES

OIL NAME

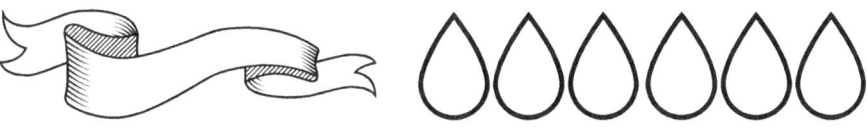

BENEFITS
_____
_____
_____
_____

NOTES
_____
_____
_____
_____

OIL NAME

BENEFITS
_____
_____
_____
_____

NOTES
_____
_____
_____
_____

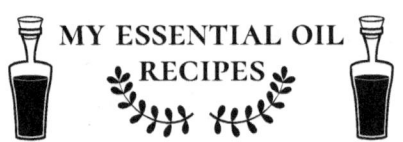

MY ESSENTIAL OIL RECIPES

OIL NAME

○○○○○○

BENEFITS
_____
_____
_____
_____

NOTES
_____
_____
_____
_____

OIL NAME

○○○○○○

BENEFITS
_____
_____
_____
_____

NOTES
_____
_____
_____
_____

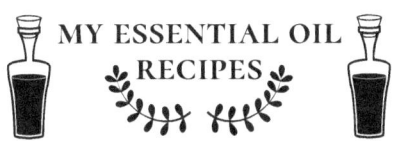
MY ESSENTIAL OIL RECIPES

OIL NAME

BENEFITS
_____
_____
_____
_____

NOTES
_____
_____
_____
_____

OIL NAME

BENEFITS
_____
_____
_____
_____

NOTES
_____
_____
_____
_____

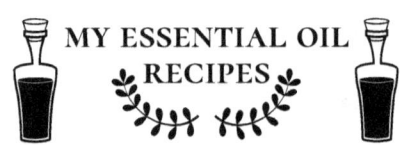
MY ESSENTIAL OIL RECIPES

OIL NAME

◯ ◯ ◯ ◯ ◯ ◯

BENEFITS
_____
_____
_____
_____

NOTES
_____
_____
_____
_____

OIL NAME

◯ ◯ ◯ ◯ ◯ ◯

BENEFITS
_____
_____
_____
_____

NOTES
_____
_____
_____
_____

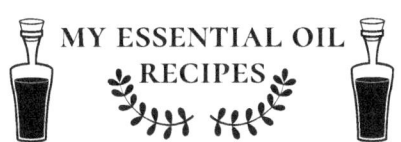
MY ESSENTIAL OIL RECIPES

OIL NAME

BENEFITS
_____
_____
_____
_____

NOTES
_____
_____
_____
_____

OIL NAME

BENEFITS
_____
_____
_____
_____

NOTES
_____
_____
_____
_____

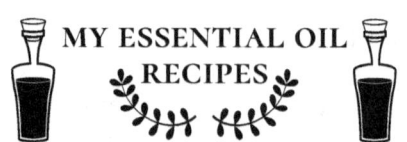
MY ESSENTIAL OIL RECIPES

OIL NAME

◊◊◊◊◊◊

BENEFITS
___
___
___
___

NOTES
___
___
___
___

OIL NAME

◊◊◊◊◊◊

BENEFITS
___
___
___
___

NOTES
___
___
___
___

www.ingramcontent.com/pod-product-compliance
Lightning Source LLC
Chambersburg PA
CBHW071409080526
44587CB00017B/3231